PLANT BASED LUPUS COOKBOOK FOR WOMEN

20 + NATURAL RECIPES TO OVERCOME FLARES, SOOTHE INFLAMMATION AND RESTORE WELLNESS.

KAREN EDMONDS

TABLE OF CONTENT

STAY HEALTHY

INTRODUCTION

The Plant-Based Lupus Cookbook emerges as a light of empowerment, developed exclusively for the resilient women traversing the maze of Lupus. Within its pages, a culinary symphony develops, providing not just recipes but also a culinary sanctuary—a celebration of health, strength, and the transformational power of plant-based life.

This cookbook is a story, a whispered promise that each ingredient has a purpose beyond flavour. Curated with precision and care, it exemplifies the concept that food can provide both health and joy. It addresses the specific requirements of women living with Lupus, guiding them through a vivid palette of anti-inflammatory miracles, nutrient-dense treasures, and delightful plant-based proteins. From the enticing appeal of Overnight Oats Varieties to the soothing warmth of Quinoa Breakfast Porridge, each dish is a brushstroke on the canvas of well-being.

However, this cookbook goes beyond the scope of a standard culinary guide. It is a kind and understanding call for women to reclaim their narratives via mindful nutrition. It promotes not only Lupus-friendly foods, but also a restored feeling of agency—a delicious path to health and self-discovery.

For any woman looking for more than just food, the Plant-Based Lupus Cookbook demonstrates the transforming power of plant-powered life. Here, in the alchemy of flavours, is a story of empowerment, a narrative in which each meal is a step towards healing and each page is a declaration of strength.

CHAPTER 1

Understanding Lupus and the Power of Plant-Based Nutrition

Lupus, a chronic autoimmune illness, presents unique problems for people affected, necessitating a sophisticated approach to diet for symptom management and general well-being. In this part, we look at the complex relationship between lupus and the transforming power of a plant-based diet.

Plant-based diets are known to have anti-inflammatory qualities, which can help manage lupus symptoms. Whole foods like fruits, vegetables, nuts, and seeds are high in antioxidants and phytochemicals, which help the body fight inflammation and recover naturally.

Balanced Nutrient Intake:

Lupus might hinder the body's capacity to absorb nutrients effectively. A plant-based diet rich in vitamins, minerals, and fibre promotes nutritional balance. This not only treats any inadequacies, but also strengthens the immune system and helps to maintain energy levels.

Gut Health and Immunity:

Plant-based diets promote a healthy gut flora, which helps regulate the immune system. A healthy stomach can improve the immune response and help treat lupus flares. Plant meals, which include prebiotics and fibre, support good gut bacteria, creating a robust digestive system.

Reduced Oxidative Stress:

Lupus can cause increased oxidative stress, leading to cell damage and worsening symptoms. Plant-based meals have an abundance of antioxidants, which help neutralise free radicals, lowering oxidative stress and contributing to cellular health.

Cardiovascular Health and Lupus:

Lupus patients are more likely to experience cardiovascular difficulties. Plant-based diets are inherently low in saturated fats and cholesterol, which promotes cardiovascular health. This food option promotes cardiovascular health, which is critical for those living with lupus.

Understanding lupus in light of the potential of plant-based diet reveals a more comprehensive approach to wellbeing. Lupus patients may fuel their bodies, ease symptoms, and begin on a road to a more vibrant and robust existence by embracing the rich tapestry of plant foods.

STAY HOPEFUL

CHAPTER 2: GETTING STARTED

Essential Ingredients

Leafy Greens:

Leafy greens such as spinach, kale and Swiss chard are essential for a plant-based diet due to their high vitamin, mineral, and antioxidant content. They improve general health and help manage inflammation.

Colorful Vegetables:

Colourful vegetables like bell peppers, carrots, and tomatoes provide a varied spectrum of nutrients. These bright options provide a wide range of antioxidants and add richness to your recipes.

Whole grains:

Choose whole grains, such as quinoa, brown rice, and oats. These grains include vital fibre, complex carbs, and a range of micronutrients that are necessary for long-term energy and digestion.

Legumes:

Plant-based protein sources include legumes such as beans, lentils, and chickpeas. They are also high in fibre, which promotes intestinal health, and make adaptable complements to soups, stews, and salads.

Nuts and seeds:

Nuts and seeds, including almonds, walnuts, chia seeds, and flaxseeds, provide omega-3 fatty acids that promote heart health and reduce inflammation. These may be sprinkled over salads, yoghurt, or eaten as snacks.

Healthy Fats:

Avocados and olive oil provide healthful fats. These fats aid in brain function, nutrient absorption, and provide a fulfilling and tasty gastronomic experience.

Kitchen Tools and Tips.

High-Quality Blender:

A high-quality blender is essential for preparing smoothies, sauces, and creamy soups. Invest in a reliable blender to easily integrate a range of fruits and vegetables into your regular diet.

Chef's Knife:

Using a sharp chef's knife improves efficiency and enjoyment of cooking. A good chef's knife is a multipurpose instrument for cutting vegetables, fruits, and herbs, assuring accuracy in your culinary endeavours.

Non-stick Pan:

Non-stick cookware reduces the need for oil, leading to a healthier cooking technique. They are perfect for sautéing vegetables, making plant-based protein substitutes, and reducing excess fat.

Food Processor:

Food processors make chopping, slicing, and mixing easier, saving time in the kitchen. It's very handy for making homemade dips, spreads, and nut-based recipes.

Steamer Basket:

Steaming is a mild cooking method that preserves the nutritional value of vegetables. A steamer basket is a useful tool for fast cooking nutrient-dense foods while retaining their natural flavours.

Fresh Herbs:

Incorporate fresh herbs into your recipes to enhance their flavour. Consider growing a small herb garden or storing a variety of widely used herbs such as basil, cilantro, and parsley for increased flavour and nutritional benefits.

Embracing a plant-based lifestyle gets easier with the correct products and kitchen utensils. By embracing these elements, you provide the groundwork for a varied and fulfilling culinary experience that benefits your overall health.

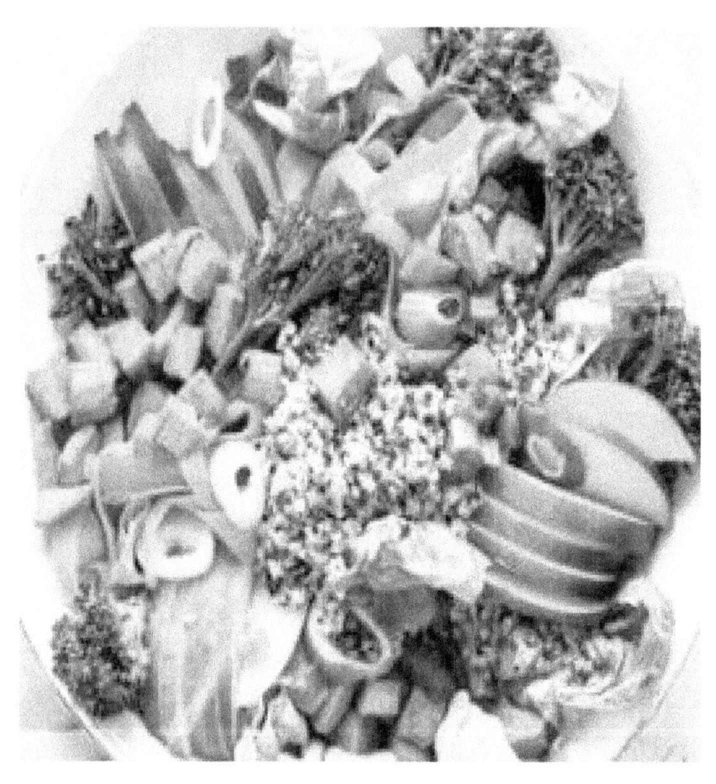

CHAPTER 3: BREAKFAST DELIGHTS

Energizing Smoothie Bowls

Ingredients:

Base:

- 1 frozen banana (peeled and sliced)
- 1 cup of mixed berries (strawberries, blueberries, raspberries)
- 1/2 cup of spinach leaves (fresh or frozen)
- 1/2 cup of unsweetened almond milk or any other plant-based milk of choice

Toppings:

- Fresh fruits, sliced (kiwi, banana, berries)
- Granola for crunch
- Chia seeds or flaxseeds for added omega-3
- Shredded coconut adds a tropical touch

- Drizzle of honey or maple syrup (optional)

Instructions:

Blend the Base:

- To make the base, mix frozen banana, berries, spinach, and almond milk in a high-speed blender. Blend until smooth and creamy. If necessary, add additional almond milk to get the desired consistency.

Prepare the toppings:

- Slice the fresh fruits and set aside. Gather granola, chia seeds, flaxseeds, and shredded coconut for the toppings.

Assemble the Bowl

- Pour the smoothie into a bowl. Level the surface with a spoon to provide an equal appearance.

Toppings:

- Arrange sliced fruits, granola, chia seeds, and shredded coconut on top of the smoothie base. This provides texture, flavour, and a wide range of nutrients.

Optional:

- Drizzle with honey or maple syrup to add sweetness to the toppings. This step is optional and can be changed according to your preferences.
- For optimal results, drink these energising smoothie bowls immediately. Grab a spoon and enjoy the delicious blend of creamy smoothie and crunchy toppings.

Nutritional Value (approx. per serving):

Calories: 300-370 kcal

Protein: 6-10g

Dietary Fiber: 12-16g

Healthy Fats: 9-13g

Carbohydrates: 52-60g

Overnight Oats Varieties

Classic Maple-Berry Bliss

Ingredients:

- 1/2 cup of rolled oats
- 1/2 cup of almond milk
- 1 tablespoon of chia seeds
- 1/2 teaspoon vanilla extract
- 1 tablespoon maple syrup
- Mixed berries (strawberries, blueberries, raspberries)
- Sliced almonds for topping

Instructions:

- Mix oats, almond milk, chia seeds, vanilla extract, and maple syrup in a jar. Stir well, refrigerate overnight. Add mixed berries and sliced almonds as toppings before serving.

Nutritional Value (approx. per serving):

Calories: 250-300 kcal

Protein: 5-7g

Dietary Fiber: 6-8g

Healthy Fats: 8-10g

Carbohydrates: 40-45g

Peanut Butter Banana Crunch

Ingredients:

- 1/2 cup of rolled oats
- 1/2 cup of coconut milk
- 1 tablespoon peanut butter
- 1/2 banana, mashed
- 1/2 teaspoon of cinnamon
- Granola for topping

Instructions:

- Combine oats, coconut milk, peanut butter, mashed banana, and cinnamon in a jar. Refrigerate overnight. To enjoy sprinkle granola on top.

Nutritional Value (approx. per serving):

Calories: 250-300 kcal

Protein: 5-7g

Dietary Fiber: 6-8g

Healthy Fats: 8-10g

Carbohydrates: 40-45g

Apple Cinnamon Delight

Ingredients:

- 1/2 cup of rolled oats
- 1/2 cup of applesauce(unsweetened)
- 1/2 cup of almond milk
- 1 tablespoon of chopped walnuts
- 1/2 teaspoon of cinnamon
- Sliced apple for topping

Instructions:

- Combine oats, applesauce, almond milk, chopped walnuts, and cinnamon in a jar. Refrigerate overnight. Before serving garnish with sliced apples.

Nutritional Value (approx. per serving):

Calories: 250-300 kcal

Protein: 5-7g

Dietary Fiber: 6-8g

Healthy Fats: 8-10g

Carbohydrates: 40-45g

Tropical Paradise

Ingredients:

- 1/2 cup of rolled oats
- 1/2 cup of pineapple juice
- 1/2 cup of coconut milk
- 1/4 cup of diced mango
- 1 tablespoon of shredded coconut
- Kiwi slices for topping

Instructions:

- Combine oats, pineapple juice, coconut milk, diced mango, and shredded coconut in a jar. Refrigerate overnight.

Place kiwi slices as topping before enjoying in a taste of the tropics.

Nutritional Value (approx. per serving):

Calories: 250-300 kcal

Protein: 5-7g

Dietary Fiber: 6-8g

Healthy Fats: 8-10g

Carbohydrates: 40-45g

Note: Nutritional values may vary based on specific ingredients and portion sizes

Quinoa Breakfast Porridge

Ingredients:

- 1/2 cup of quinoa, washed
- 1 cup almond milk (or any plant-based milk of choice)
- 1/2 teaspoon of vanilla extract
- 1 tablespoon maple syrup or honey
- 1/4 teaspoon of ground cinnamon

- Fresh berries (strawberries, blueberries, raspberries) for topping
- Chopped nuts (almonds, walnuts) for garnish
- Sliced banana for added sweetness (optional)

Instructions:

Rinse Quinoa:

- Rinse quinoa under cold water to eliminate any bitterness.

Cook Quinoa:

- To cook quinoa, add almond milk to a pot. Bring to a boil, then decrease heat to low, cover, and cook for 15-20 minutes, or until the quinoa is tender and most of the liquid has been absorbed.

Add flavour and sweetness:

- To add flavour and sweetness, stir in vanilla essence, maple syrup (or honey), and ground cinnamon. Adjust the sweetness to your preference.

Serve:

- To serve, transfer the quinoa porridge to a bowl. If preferred, add fresh berries, chopped almonds, and sliced banana.
- To enhance flavour and texture, consider adding toppings like almond butter or coconut flakes.

Nutritional Value (approx. per serving):

Calories: 350-400 kcal

Protein: 10-12g

Dietary Fiber: 6-8g

Healthy Fats: 8-10g

Carbohydrates: 60-70g

CHAPTER 4: LUNCH IDEAS

Ingredients:

For the Salad:

- 1 can (15 oz) chickpeas, washed and drained
- 1 cup of cherry tomatoes, halved
- 1 cucumber, finely diced
- 1 red bell pepper, diced
- 1/2 red onion, finely chopped
- 1/4 cup of Kalamata olives, sliced
- 1/4 cup of fresh parsley, cut

For the Dressing:

- 3 tablespoons of extra virgin olive oil
- 1 tablespoon of red wine vinegar
- 1 teaspoon of Dijon mustard
- 1 clove of minced garlic
- Salt and pepper to taste

Optional Additions:

- Feta cheese crumbles
- Avocado slices

Instructions:

Prepare Chickpeas:

- Washed and drain chickpeas thoroughly. If time permits, blot them dry with a clean kitchen towel to get a sharper texture.

Cut and Dice Vegetables:

- In a large mixing bowl, add cherry tomatoes, cucumber, red bell pepper, red onion, olives, and fresh parsley.

Assemble Salad:

- To assemble the salad, combine chickpeas with vegetables in a dish.

Make the Dressing:

- To make the dressing, mix olive oil, red wine vinegar, Dijon mustard, minced garlic, salt, and pepper in a small bowl. Adjust the seasoning to your liking.

Mix and Toss:

- Toss the salad ingredients and pour the dressing on top. Gently mix everything together until evenly covered.

Marinate:

- To marinate, cover the salad and refrigerate for at least 30 minutes. This also allows the chickpeas to absorb the dressing.

Serve:

- Before serving, give the salad a last spin. Optionally, top with feta cheese crumbles and avocado slices for an added layer of creaminess and richness.

Nutritional Value (approx. per serving):

Calories: 300-350 kcal

Protein: 10-12g

Dietary Fiber: 8-10g

Healthy Fats: 15-18g

Carbohydrates: 35-40g

Ingredients:

For the Roasted Vegetables:

- 1 zucchini, finely sliced
- 1 red bell pepper, sliced
- 1 yellow bell pepper, sliced
- 1 red onion, finely sliced
- 1 cup cherry tomatoes, halved
- 2 tablespoons of olive oil
- 1 teaspoon of dried oregano
- Salt and pepper to taste

For the Wrap Assembly:

- Whole wheat or spinach tortillas
- Hummus or your preferred spread
- Spinach leaves, fresh
- Feta cheese crumbles (optional)
- Balsamic glaze for drizzling (optional)

Instructions:

Preheat the Oven:

- Preheat the oven to 400°F (200°C).

Prepare Vegetables:

- In a large mixing bowl, add zucchini, red and yellow peppers, red onion and cherry tomatoes. Drizzle with olive oil, then add the dried oregano, salt, and pepper. Toss the vegetables until uniformly coated.

Roast vegetables:

- To roast vegetables, spread seasoned vegetables on a baking sheet lined with parchment paper. Roast in a preheated oven for 20-25 minutes, or until the vegetables are soft and faintly caramelised.

Assemble wraps:

- To assemble wraps, warm the tortillas slightly. Spread a liberal amount of hummus or your favourite spread onto each tortilla.

Layer with Spinach and Roasted vegetables:

- Place a handful of fresh spinach leaves on each tortilla, then a piece of roasted vegetables.

Optional:

- Sprinkle crumbled feta cheese over vegetables for a creamy touch.

Optional:

- Drizzle balsamic glaze over vegetables to enhance flavour.

Wrap and serve:

- To wrap and serve, fold the tortilla's sides and roll firmly. Divide in half diagonally and serve immediately.

Nutritional Value (approx. per serving):

Calories: 350-400 kcal

Protein: 8-10g

Dietary Fiber: 8-10g

Healthy Fats: 15-18g

Carbohydrates: 45-50g

Ingredients:

- 1 cup of dried brown or green lentils, washed and drained
- 2 medium sweet potatoes, peeled and diced
- 1 onion, finely chopped
- 3 cloves of minced garlic
- 1 can (14 oz) of diced tomatoes, undrained
- 4 cups of vegetable broth
- 1 teaspoon of ground cumin
- 1 teaspoon of ground coriander
- 1/2 teaspoon of smoked paprika
- 1/2 teaspoon of turmeric
- Salt and pepper to taste
- 2 cups of kale or spinach, cut
- 1 lemon, juiced
- Fresh cilantro for garnish (optional)

Instructions:

Prepare Lentils:

- Rinse lentils under cold water and drain.

Sauté Onion and Garlic:

- In a large saucepan, cook chopped onion and minced garlic over medium heat until softened.

Add sweet potatoes:

- To add sweet potatoes, dice them and stir in the saucepan for a few minutes.

Season:

- To season, sprinkle cumin, coriander, smoked paprika, turmeric, salt, and pepper over the vegetables. Stir until evenly coated.

Combine Lentils and Tomatoes:

- To combine lentils with tomatoes, rinse them and add a can of diced tomatoes with juice to the saucepan. Mix thoroughly.

Pour in Vegetable Broth:

- Add vegetables broth and bring to a boil. Once boiling, lower the heat to low, cover, and allow it simmer for 25-30 minutes, or until the lentils and sweet potatoes are cooked.

Add Greens and Lemon Juice:

- To add greens and lemon juice, stir in chopped kale or spinach and wilt it into the stew. Squeeze the juice of one lemon into the saucepan and adjust the acidity to taste.

Adjust Seasoning:

- Taste and adjust seasoning as required. If desired, season with more salt, pepper, or spices.

Serve:

- To serve, ladle the stew into bowls and top with fresh cilantro. Serve hot.

Nutritional Value (approx. per serving):

Calories: 300-350 kcal

Protein: 15-18g

Dietary Fiber: 10-12g

Healthy Fats: 2-4g

Carbohydrates: 55-60g

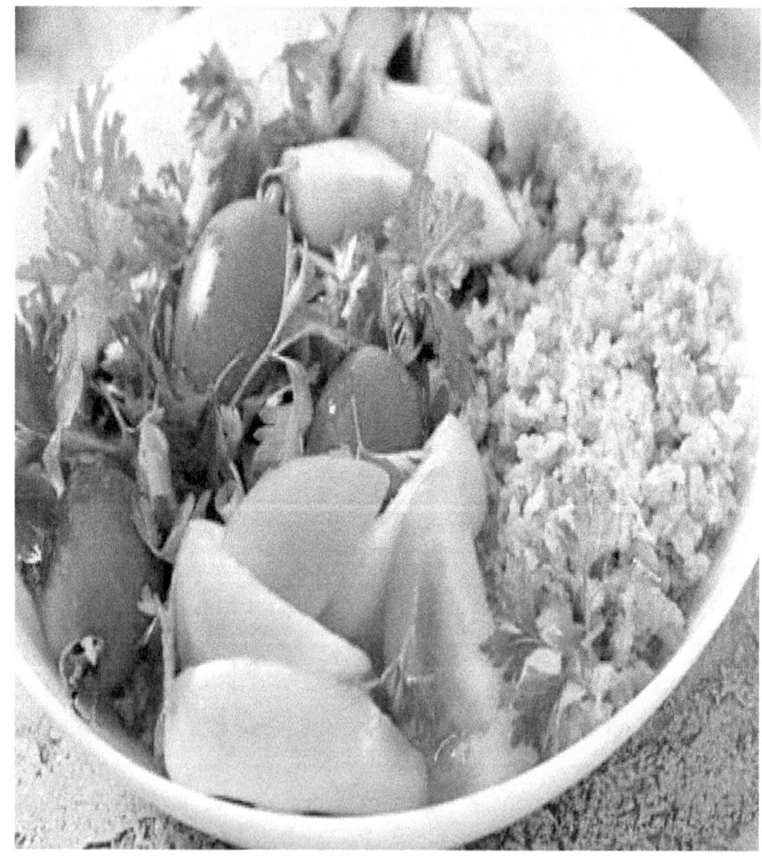

CHAPTER 5: NOURISHING DINNER RECIPES

Ingredients:

- 1 1/2 cups of Arborio rice (or any other kind of risotto rice)
- 1 cup cremini or button mushrooms, chopped
- 2 cups of chopped fresh spinach
- 1 onion, finely chopped
- 3 cloves of minced garlic
- 1/2 cup dry white wine (optional)
- 4 cups of vegetable broth, kept warm
- 1/2 cup of grated Parmesan cheese
- 2 tablespoons butter
- 2 tablespoons of olive oil
- Salt and black pepper to taste
- Fresh parsley for garnish

Instructions:

Prepare Mushroom and Spinach:

- To prepare the mushrooms and spinach, heat 1 tablespoon olive oil in a big skillet or pan over medium heat. Sauté the mushrooms until they lose moisture and turn golden brown. Add the chopped spinach and simmer until wilted. Place aside.

Sauté Onion and Garlic:

- Sauté onion and garlic in the same pan with the remaining olive oil. Sauté the chopped onions until transparent, then add the minced garlic and fry until aromatic.

Toast Arborio Rice:

- To toast Arborio rice, add it to a skillet and stir continually for a few minutes, until the edges become translucent.

Deglaze with Wine (Optional):

- To deglaze the pan, add white wine (optional) and stir continually until the liquid evaporates.

Add Broth:

- Begin adding heated vegetable broth, one ladle at a time, stirring frequently. Allow the liquid to soak before adding the next ladle. Continue cooking the rice until it is creamy and al dente.

Integrate Mushroom and Spinach:

- Fold in sautéed mushrooms and spinach to the almost cooked rice. Let the flavours merge for a few minutes.

Finish with Butter and Cheese:

- To finish, stir in butter and grated Parmesan cheese. Season with salt and black pepper to taste. Continue stirring until the risotto has a creamy consistency.

Garnish and Serve:

- Remove from heat, sprinkle with fresh parsley, and serve right away.

Nutritional Value (approx. per serving):

Calories: 400-450 kcal

Protein: 8-10g

Dietary Fiber: 3-5g

Healthy Fats: 14-16g

Carbohydrates: 60-65g

Walnut-Crusted Eggplant Parmesan

Ingredients:

For the Eggplant:

- 2 big eggplants, finely and thinly sliced
- Salt for sweating the eggplant
- 2 cups of breadcrumbs (whole wheat preferably)
- 1 cup of walnuts, finely chopped
- 1 cup of grated Parmesan cheese

- 3 eggs, beaten
- 1 cup of all-purpose flour
- Olive oil for frying

For the Assembly:

- 2 cups of marinara sauce
- 2 cups of shredded mozzarella cheese
- Fresh basil leaves for garnish
- Additional Parmesan for serving

Instructions:

Prepare Eggplant Slices:

- To prepare eggplant slices, thinly slice the eggplants. Sprinkle salt on both sides of each slice and let to sweat for about 30 minutes. To eliminate any extra moisture, pat dry with paper towels.

Prepare Breading Station:

- Create a breading station with three shallow dishes. Fill one with flour, the other with beaten eggs, and the third with breadcrumbs, chopped walnuts, and grated Parmesan cheese.

Bread the Eggplant:

- To bread eggplant, dredge in flour, dip in beaten eggs, then coat with breadcrumb-walnut mixture. Press lightly to adhere.

Fry Eggplant Slices:

- To fry eggplant slices, heat olive oil in a large pan over medium heat. Fry the breaded aubergine till golden brown on both sides. Place them on a dish lined with paper towels to absorb any extra oil.

Preheat Oven:

- Preheat oven to 375°F (190°C).

Assemble Eggplant Parmesan:

- To make Eggplant Parmesan: In a baking dish, pour a thin layer of marinara. Layer fried eggplant slices on top, then sprinkle with shredded mozzarella. Repeat the layers until all of the ingredients have been utilised, then top with a layer of cheese.

Bake:

- Bake in a preheated oven for 25-30 minutes, or until cheese is melted and bubbling.

Garnish and Serve:

- After removing from the oven, sprinkle with fresh basil leaves and serve hot. Optional: Top with more Parmesan cheese.

Nutritional Value (approx. per serving):

Calories: 400-450 kcal

Protein: 15-18g

Dietary Fiber: 6-8g

Healthy Fats: 20-25g

Carbohydrates: 40-45g

Turmeric Infused Cauliflower Rice

Ingredients:

- 1 medium-sized cauliflower head, washed and dried
- 2 tablespoons of olive oil or coconut oil
- 1 teaspoon of turmeric powder
- 1/2 teaspoon ground cumin
- 1/2 teaspoon of paprika (optional for added depth of flavor)
- Salt and black pepper to taste
- Fresh cilantro or parsley for garnish

Instructions:

Prepare the Cauliflower:

- To prepare the cauliflower, remove the leaves and stalk, then cut it into florets. Using a food processor, pulse the florets until they have the texture of rice.

Sauté the Cauliflower Rice:

- To sauté the cauliflower rice, heat olive oil in a large pan over medium heat. Add the cauliflower rice and cook for 3-4 minutes, stirring often.

Add Turmeric and Spices:

- Sprinkle turmeric powder, ground cumin, and paprika over cauliflower rice. Continue to sauté, making sure the spices cover the rice evenly.

Season with Salt and Pepper:

- Season rice with salt and black pepper to taste. Adjust the seasoning to your liking.

Cook Until Soft:

- Cook cauliflower rice for a further 4-5 minutes until soft and slightly firm. Be careful not to overcook cauliflower rice, since it might turn mushy.

Garnish and Serve:

- To serve, remove from heat and add fresh cilantro or parsley as garnish.

Serve immediately as a vibrant and savoury side dish.

Nutritional Value (approx. per serving):

Calories: 50-60 kcal

Protein: 2-3g

Dietary Fiber: 3-4g

Healthy Fats: 4-5g

Carbohydrates: 5-6g

CHAPTER 6: SNACKS AND APPETIZERS

Ingredients:

- 1 ripe avocado, peeled and pitted
- 1 can (15 oz) chickpeas, rinsed and drained
- 2 cloves of minced garlic
- 3 tablespoons of tahini
- 3 tablespoons of extra virgin olive oil
- 1 lemon, juiced
- 1/2 teaspoon of ground cumin
- Salt and black pepper to taste
- Fresh cilantro or parsley for garnish
- Optional toppings: drizzle of olive oil, red pepper flakes

Instructions:

Combine Ingredients:

- In a food processor, add ripe avocado, chickpeas, garlic, tahini, olive oil, lemon juice, cumin, salt, and pepper.

Blend Until Smooth:

- Blend all items until smooth and creamy. You may need to scrape the sides of the food processor to achieve even mixing.

Adjust Seasoning:

- Taste the dip and adjust seasoning as required. Adjust the seasoning with extra salt, pepper, or lemon juice as desired.

Garnish:

- To garnish, transfer the avocado hummus dip to a serving dish. Sprinkle with fresh cilantro or parsley and, if wanted, sprinkle with olive oil. To add a bit of spice, sprinkle with red pepper flakes.

Serve:

- Serve this dip with pita chips, chopped vegetables, or whole-grain crackers.

Nutritional Value (approx. per serving):

Calories: 150-180 kcal

Protein: 4-6g

Dietary Fiber: 5-7g

Healthy Fats: 10-12g

Carbohydrates: 10-12g

Baked Sweet Potato Fries

Ingredients:

- 2 big sweet potatoes, peeled and cut into small sizes (for fries)
- 2 tablespoons of olive oil
- 1 teaspoon of paprika
- 1/2 teaspoon of garlic powder
- 1/2 teaspoon of onion powder
- 1/2 teaspoon of cayenne pepper (modify to taste)
- Salt and black pepper to taste

- 2 tablespoons of corn starch (optional for added crispiness)
- Fresh parsley for garnish (optional)

Instructions:

Preheat the Oven:

- Preheat the oven to 425°F (220°C) and prepare a baking sheet with parchment paper.

Prepare Sweet Potatoes:

- To prepare sweet potatoes, peel and cut them into uniform fries of equal thickness to ensure consistent baking.

Coat with Olive Oil and Spices:

- To season sweet potato fries, combine olive oil, paprika, garlic powder, onion powder, cayenne pepper, salt, and black pepper in a big bowl. If you want more crispiness, add cornflour and stir until uniformly coated.

Arrange on Baking Sheet:

- Arrange seasoned sweet potato fries in a single layer on a baking sheet to ensure uniform cooking.

Bake:

- Bake fries in a preheated oven for 20-25 minutes, turning halfway through to maintain even crispness. Adjust the cooking time to get the appropriate amount of crispiness.

Serve:

- To serve, remove the sweet potato fries from the oven after they have turned golden brown and crispy. Garnish with fresh parsley if preferred and serve immediately.

Nutritional Value (approx. per serving):

Calories: 150-180 kcal

Dietary Fiber: 4-6g

Healthy Fats: 6-8g

Carbohydrates: 25-30g

Zesty Guacamole with Vegetable Sticks

Ingredients:

For Guacamole:

- 3 ripe avocados, peeled and pitted
- 1 small red onion, finely sliced
- 2 tomatoes, finely diced
- 1-2 cloves of minced garlic
- 2 limes, juiced
- 1/4 cup of fresh cilantro, chopped
- Salt and black pepper to taste
- Optional: Jalapeño, diced (for a spicy kick)

For Vegetable Sticks:

- Carrot sticks
- Cucumber sticks
- Bell pepper strips (assorted colors)
- Celery sticks

Instructions:

Prepare Guacamole:

- To make guacamole, mash ripe avocados in a large basin with a fork until smooth and slightly chunky.

Add Vegetables:

- To add vegetables, mix in finely chopped red onion, diced tomatoes, minced garlic, lime juice, and cilantro to the mashed avocado. For a spicy kick, add diced jalapeño.

Season:

- Season guacamole with salt and black pepper. Adjust the seasoning to your liking.

Mix Well:

- Mix well by gently folding in all ingredients. To keep a chunky texture, avoid overmixing.

Prepare Vegetables Sticks:

- To prepare veggie sticks, wash and chop a variety of fresh vegetables into sticks. Carrot sticks, cucumber sticks, bell pepper strips, and celery sticks all work nicely.

Serve:

- To serve, set a serving bowl of Zesty Guacamole in the centre of a plate. Surround the guacamole with a colourful selection of vegetable spears.

Optional garnish:

- Add cilantro and lime wedges to guacamole.

Enjoy:

- Enjoy this savoury dip with crisp, refreshing vegetable sticks.

Nutritional Value (approx. per serving):

Calories: 150-180 kcal

Dietary Fiber: 8-10g

Healthy Fats: 12-15g

Carbohydrates: 12-15g

CHAPTER 7: SWEETS AND TREATS

Berry Bliss Chia Pudding

Ingredients:

For Chia Pudding:

- 1/4 cup of chia seeds
- 1 cup of almond milk (or any plant-based milk of choice)
- 1-2 tablespoons of maple syrup or honey (adjust to taste)
- 1/2 teaspoon of vanilla extract

For Berry Compote:

- 1 cup of mixed berries (strawberries, blueberries, raspberries)
- 1-2 tablespoons of maple syrup or honey
- 1 tablespoon water
- 1/2 teaspoon of lemon juice

For Toppings:

- Fresh berries for garnish
- Greek yogurt (optional)
- Granola (optional)
- Mint leaves for garnish (optional)

Instructions:

Prepare Chia Pudding:

- To make Chia Pudding, combine chia seeds, almond milk, maple syrup or honey and vanilla essence in a bowl. Make sure the chia seeds are properly mixed. Allow it to settle for a few minutes, then whisk again to prevent clumping. Refrigerate for at least 2-3 hours, preferably overnight, to allow the chia seeds to absorb the liquid and form a pudding-like texture.

Make Berry Compote:

- To make berry compote, blend berries, maple syrup or honey, water, and lemon juice in a saucepan. Cook over medium heat, stirring regularly, until the berries have broken down and the mixture thickens into a compote. Remove from heat and allow to cool.

Prepare the Pudding:

- Add a layer of chia pudding to serving glasses or bowls. Add a layer of berry compote on top.

Repeat Layers:

- Repeat layering until glasses are full, then top with berry compote.

Refrigerate:

- Refrigerate the Berry Bliss Chia Pudding for an extra 30 minutes to enable flavours to mingle and solidify.

Toppings:

- Optional toppings include fresh berries, Greek yoghurt, granola, and mint leaves.

Nutritional Value (approx. per serving):

Calories: 250-300 kcal

Protein: 5-7g

Dietary Fiber: 10-12g

Healthy Fats: 10-12g

Carbohydrates: 35-40g

Banana-Oat Cookies

Ingredients:

- 2 ripe bananas, mashed
- 1 cup of rolled oats
- 1/4 cup of almond butter or peanut butter
- 1/4 cup of raisins or dark chocolate chips (optional)
- 1 teaspoon of vanilla extract
- 1/2 teaspoon of cinnamon
- Pinch of salt

Instructions:

Preheat the Oven:

- Preheat oven to 350°F (180°C). Line baking sheet with parchment paper.

Mash Bananas:

- In a mixing basin, mash ripe bananas with a fork until smooth.

Include Oats and Nut Butter:

- Add rolled oats, almond or peanut butter, vanilla essence, cinnamon, and salt to mashed bananas. Stir until all ingredients are thoroughly blended.

Add Raisins or Chocolate Chips (Optional):

- Fold in raisins or dark chocolate chips for added sweetness and texture to cookie batter.

Scoop and Flatten:

- To make the cookies, use a spoon or cookie scoop to put spoonfuls onto a baking sheet. Flatten as needed. Flatten each cookie gently using the back of a spoon or your fingertips.

Bake:

- To bake, preheat the oven and bake for 12-15 minutes until golden brown on the edges.

Allow to cool:

- Allow cookies to cool on baking sheet for a few minutes before moving them to a wire rack to finish cooling.

Preserve:

- After cooling, refrigerate the Banana-Oat Cookies in an airtight container. They can be preserved at room temperature for a couple of days or refrigerated for extended freshness.

Nutritional Value (approx. per serving):

Calories: 90-120 kcal per cookie

Protein: 2-3g

Dietary Fiber: 2-3g

Healthy Fats: 4-6g

Carbohydrates: 12-15g

Dark Chocolate Avocado Mousse

Ingredients:

- 2 ripe avocados, peeled and pitted
- 1/2 cup of dark chocolate chips or chopped dark chocolate (70% cocoa or higher)
- 1/4 cup of cocoa powder (unsweetened)
- 1/4 cup of maple syrup
- 1 teaspoon of vanilla extract
- Pinch of salt
- Optional toppings: Fresh berries, mint leaves, or a sprinkle of cocoa powder

Instructions:

Melt Chocolate:

- To melt chocolate, use a double boiler or microwave in short bursts. Stir until smooth and place aside to cool slightly.

Blend Avocados:

- In a blender or food processor, add ripe avocados, melted chocolate, unsweetened cocoa powder, maple syrup, vanilla extract, and salt.

Blend till smooth:

- Blend until smooth and creamy. Scrape down the sides of the blender or food processor as required to produce an equal mix.

Modify:

- Taste the mousse and adjust as needed. For a sweeter flavour, add extra maple syrup.

Refrigerate:

- After chilling, serve the Dark Chocolate Avocado Mousse in glasses or bowls. Cover and refrigerate for at least 1-2 hours to let the mousse firm.

Serve:

- To serve, decorate the mousse with fresh berries, mint leaves, or chocolate powder as preferred.

Nutritional Value (approx. per serving):

Calories: 150-180 kcal

Protein: 2-3g

Dietary Fiber: 5-7g

Healthy Fats: 10-12g

Carbohydrates: 15-20g

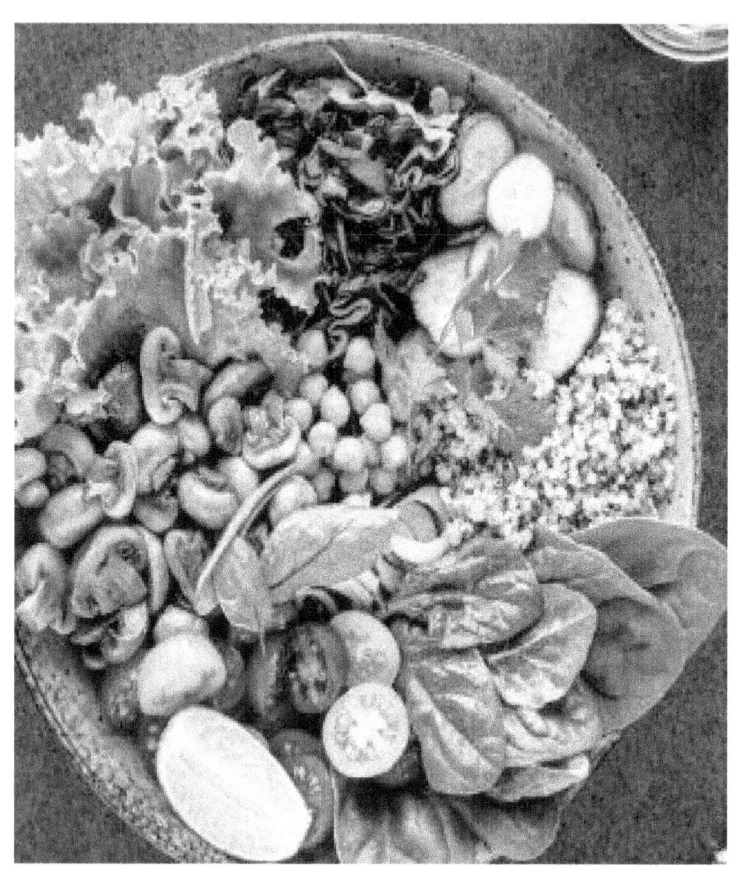

CHAPTER 8: WELLNESS BEVERAGES

Anti-Inflammatory Golden Milk

Ingredients:

- 1 cup of almond milk, unsweetened (or any plant-based milk)
- 1 teaspoon of ground turmeric
- 1/2 teaspoon of crushed cinnamon
- 1/4 teaspoon of powdered ginger (or grated fresh ginger)
- 1/4 teaspoon of ground cardamom
- Pinch of black pepper (improves turmeric absorption)
- 1 tablespoon of maple syrup or honey (adjust to taste)
- 1/2 teaspoon of coconut oil (optional)
- Optional: Dash of ground nutmeg or a cinnamon stick for garnish

Instructions:

Warm the Milk:

- Heat the almond milk in a small saucepan over a medium heat until warm but not boiling.

Add the Spices:

- Add ground turmeric, cinnamon, ginger, cardamom, and black pepper to heated milk.

Whisk:

- To cook, whisk together the ingredients and simmer on low heat for 5-7 minutes. Stir occasionally to ensure that the spices are fully absorbed.

Sweeten and Include Fat:

- To sweeten and add fat, add maple syrup or honey to the golden milk. Add coconut oil for a hint of healthful fat and creaminess. Continue to boil for another 1-2 minutes.

- Strain golden milk to remove spices. This step is optional since some individuals prefer the feel and advantages of eating entire spices.
- To serve, pour the Anti-Inflammatory Golden Milk into a cup. Garnish with a pinch of ground nutmeg or a cinnamon stick, if preferred.

Enjoy:

- Enjoy the calming flavours of this warm, anti-inflammatory beverage.

Nutritional Value (approx. per serving):

Calories: 80-100 kcal

Dietary Fiber: 1-2g

Healthy Fats: 2-3g

Carbohydrates: 15-20g

Refreshing Cucumber Mint Lemonade

Ingredients:

- 1 big cucumber, peeled and finey sliced
- 1/2 cup of fresh mint leaves
- 1 cup freshly of squeezed lemon juice (about 5 lemons)
- 1/2 cup of granulated sugar or sweetener of your choice (adjust to taste)
- 4 cups of cold water
- Ice cubes for serving
- Lemon slices and mint sprigs for garnish

Instructions:

Prepare Cucumber and Mint:

- Peel and slice the cucumber into rounds. Wash the mint leaves very well.

Blend Cucumber and mint:

- In a blender, mix cucumber slices and mint leaves. Blend until smooth.

Strain (Optional):

- For a smoother consistency, strain the cucumber-mint puree through a fine mesh sieve or cheesecloth to remove juice. This stage is optional, however some individuals prefer the texture and extra fibre.

Add Lemon juice and Sugar:

- In a pitcher, add freshly squeezed lemon juice and granulated sugar. Stir vigorously until the sugar has dissolved.

Mix Ingredients:

- To prepare, combine cucumber-mint puree, lemon juice, and sugar in a pitcher. Mix thoroughly.

Add cold water:

- Pour cold water into the pitcher and swirl to mix all contents.

- Refrigerate the pitcher for at least 1-2 hours to let the flavours mingle.

Serve:

- Place ice cubes in glasses and pour Refreshing Cucumber Mint Lemonade over them. Garnish with lemon slices and mint sprigs.

Nutritional Value (approx. per serving):

Calories: 80-100 kcal

Dietary Fiber: 1-2g

Carbohydrates: 20-25g

Vitamin C: 30-40% of the daily recommended intake

Green Tea Elixir

Ingredients:

- 2 green tea bags or 2 teaspoons loose green tea leaves
- 2 cups of hot water (not boiling)
- 1 tablespoon of honey (adjust to taste)

- 1 lemon, juiced
- 1/2 teaspoon of freshly grated ginger
- Ice cubes for serving
- Lemon slices and mint leaves for garnish (optional)

Instructions:

Brew Green Tea:

- To brew green tea, place tea bags or loose leaves in a heatproof container or teapot. Pour boiling water over the tea and steep it for 2-3 minutes. To maintain the delicate flavour of green tea, avoid boiling water.

Strain or Remove Tea bags:

- To remove loose tea leaves from the liquid, either remove the tea bags or filter them. Allow the green tea to cool to room temperature.

Include Honey and Ginger:

- Stir add honey and finely grated ginger to the green tea. Adjust the sweetness to your liking.

Add Lemon juice:

- To add lemon juice, squeeze one lemon into the green tea mixture. Stir thoroughly to mix the flavours.

Refrigerate:

- Refrigerate the Green Tea Elixir for at least 30 minutes to 1 hour.

Serve over ice:

- Add ice cubes to glasses and pour cold Green Tea Elixir over them.

Garnish:

- Optional garnishes include lemon slices and mint leaves for a colourful and fresh look.

Nutritional Value (approx. per serving):

Calories: 20-30 kcal

Antioxidants: Green tea is rich in antioxidants, such as catechins, which have potential health benefits.

Vitamin C: Lemon juice provides a dose of vitamin C, contributing to immune health.

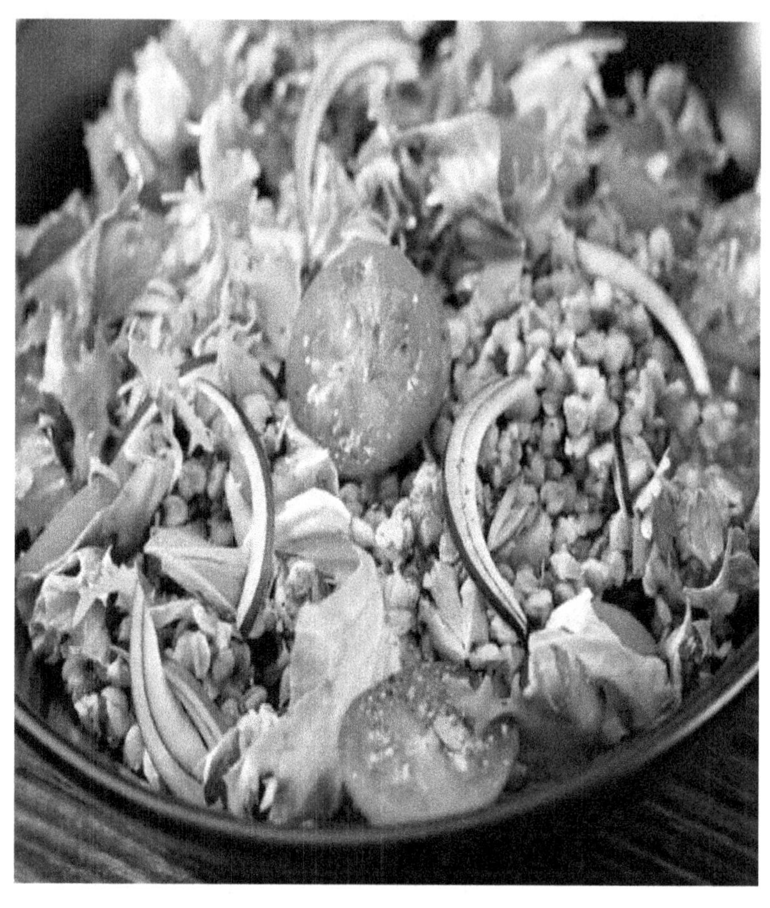

CHAPTER 9: 10-DAY MEAL PLAN

Breakfast: Quinoa Breakfast Porridge with berries and almond milk.

Lunch: Lentil and Vegetable Soup with a side of mixed greens.

Dinner: Roasted Vegetable Wraps with hummus in whole-grain tortillas.

Breakfast: Energizing Smoothie Bowl with spinach, banana, berries, and plant-based protein.

Lunch: Colorful Chickpea Salad with a variety of vegetables and a lemon-tahini dressing.

Dinner: Quinoa-Stuffed Bell Peppers with a side of steamed broccoli.

Breakfast: Overnight Oats with chia seeds, almond milk, and topped with sliced kiwi and nuts.

Lunch: Avocado Hummus Dip with veggie sticks and whole-grain crackers.

Dinner: Lentil and Sweet Potato Stew served over brown rice.

Breakfast: Berry Bliss Chia Pudding topped with sliced almonds.

Lunch: Spinach and Mushroom Risotto made with arborio rice and nutritional yeast.

Dinner: Walnut-Crusted Eggplant Parmesan with a side of quinoa.

Breakfast: Green Smoothie with kale, pineapple, mango, and coconut water.

Lunch: Chickpea and Quinoa Buddha Bowl with roasted vegetables and a tahini dressing.

Dinner: Colorful Chickpea Curry with cauliflower rice.

Breakfast: Turmeric Infused Cauliflower Rice Bowl with sautéed greens and avocado.

Lunch: Baked Sweet Potato Fries with a side of black bean and corn salsa.

Dinner: Zesty Lentil and Vegetable Stir-Fry with brown rice.

Breakfast: Banana-Oat Cookies made with mashed banana, oats, and nuts.

Lunch: Mediterranean Chickpea Salad with tomatoes, cucumber, olives, and a lemon dressing.

Dinner: Quinoa and Vegetable Stir-Fry with tofu and a ginger-soy sauce.

Breakfast: Chia Seed Pudding made with almond milk, topped with sliced strawberries and a drizzle of agave syrup.

Lunch: Quinoa and Black Bean Salad with cherry tomatoes, corn, and a cilantro-lime dressing.

Dinner: Stuffed Portobello Mushrooms with a mixture of quinoa, spinach, and diced tomatoes.

Day 9:

Breakfast: Green Tea Elixir with a slice of whole-grain toast topped with avocado.

Lunch: Vegan Caesar Salad with chickpea croutons and a creamy cashew-based dressing.

Dinner: Sweet Potato and Black Bean Enchiladas with a side of guacamole.

Day 10:

Breakfast: Smoothie Bowl with kale, mango, banana, and a sprinkle of hemp seeds.

Lunch: Mediterranean Stuffed Bell Peppers with quinoa, olives, and artichokes.

Dinner: Lentil and Vegetable Curry served over basmati rice.

Snack Ideas (Based on your choice):

Sliced cucumber with hummus

Fresh fruit (grapes, apple slices, or a pear)

Mixed nuts and seeds

Rice cakes with guacamole

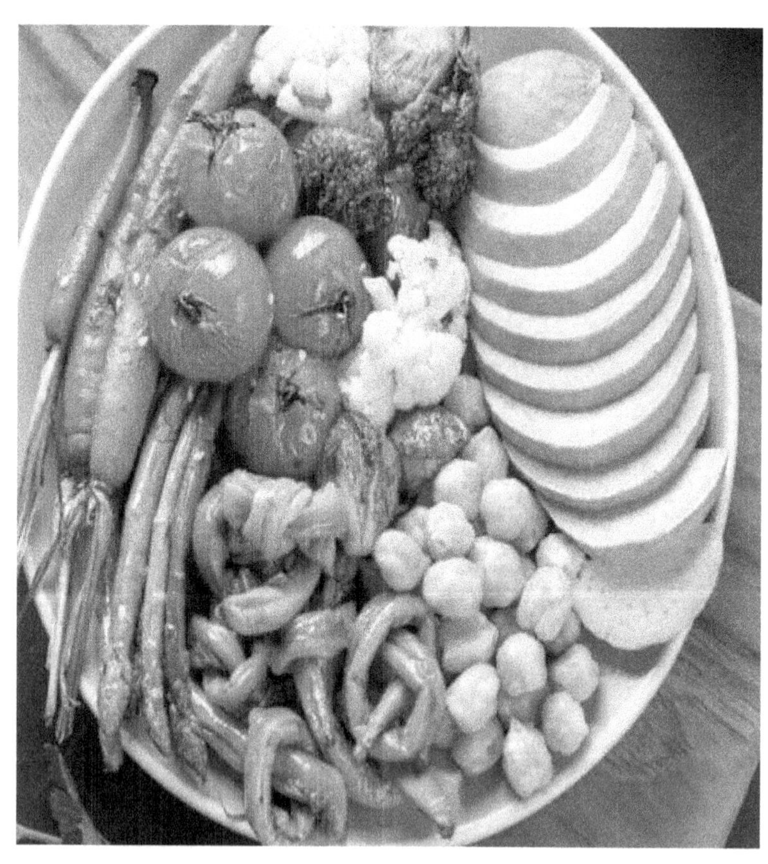

CHAPTER 10:
CONCLUSION

Finally, adopting a plant-based Lupus cookbook designed specifically for women provides a holistic approach to nutrition, emphasising anti-inflammatory and nutrient-dense components that may improve health and well-being. By including a variety of colourful fruits and vegetables, healthy grains, legumes, and plant-based proteins, this cookbook attempts to deliver a broad range of flavours and textures while keeping to Lupus-friendly principles. The recipes in this collection have been deliberately developed to meet the nutritional needs of women with Lupus, with an emphasis on antioxidants, critical vitamins, and anti-inflammatory characteristics.

Furthermore, the plant-based Lupus cookbook aims to inspire women to take control of their health by making thoughtful and deliberate eating choices. The use of substances recognised for their possible anti-inflammatory and immune-supportive properties may lead to a sense of empowerment and control over one's health. As a tool for developing good behaviours, this cookbook enables women with Lupus to discover the rich world of plant-based cuisine, building a positive relationship with food that not only tastes wonderful but also helps them on their path to healing.

Finally, the plant-based Lupus cookbook for women acts as a guide, offering not only healthy dishes but also inspiration for developing a lifestyle centred on balanced nutrition, self-care, and resilience in the face of health issues.

STAY HEALTHY!

BONUS

MEAL PLANNER

*D*AILY

DATE

BREAKFAST

NOTES

LUNCH

SNACK

ITEMS LIST

DINNER

MEAL PLANNER

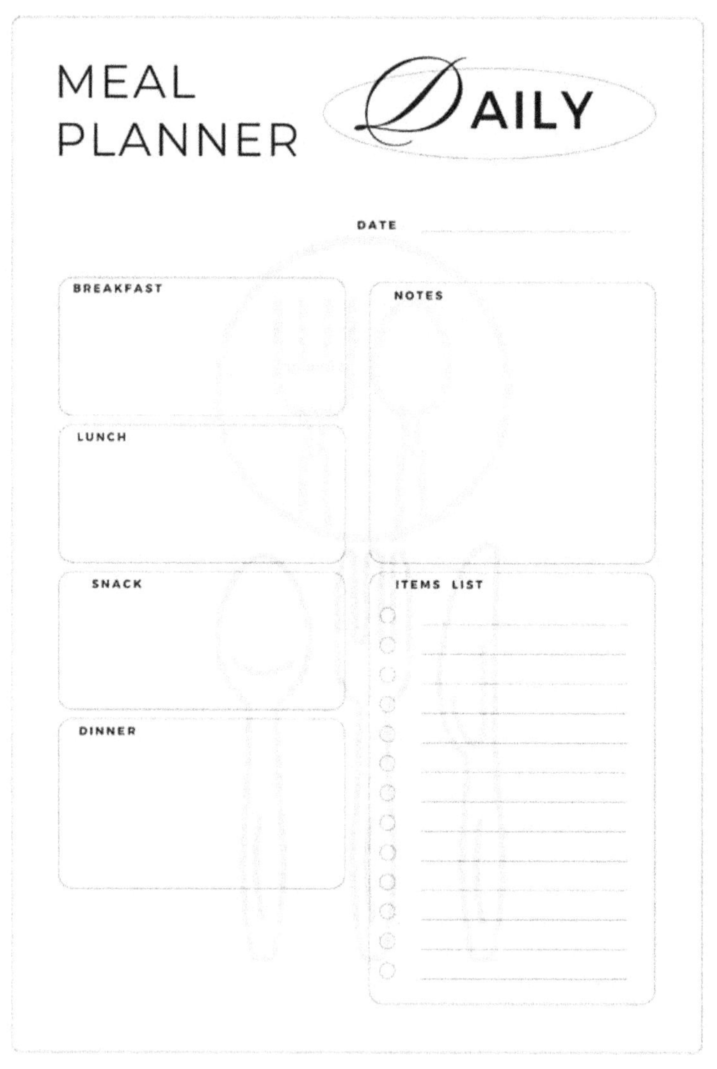

DAILY

DATE

BREAKFAST

LUNCH

SNACK

DINNER

NOTES

ITEMS LIST

MEAL PLANNER

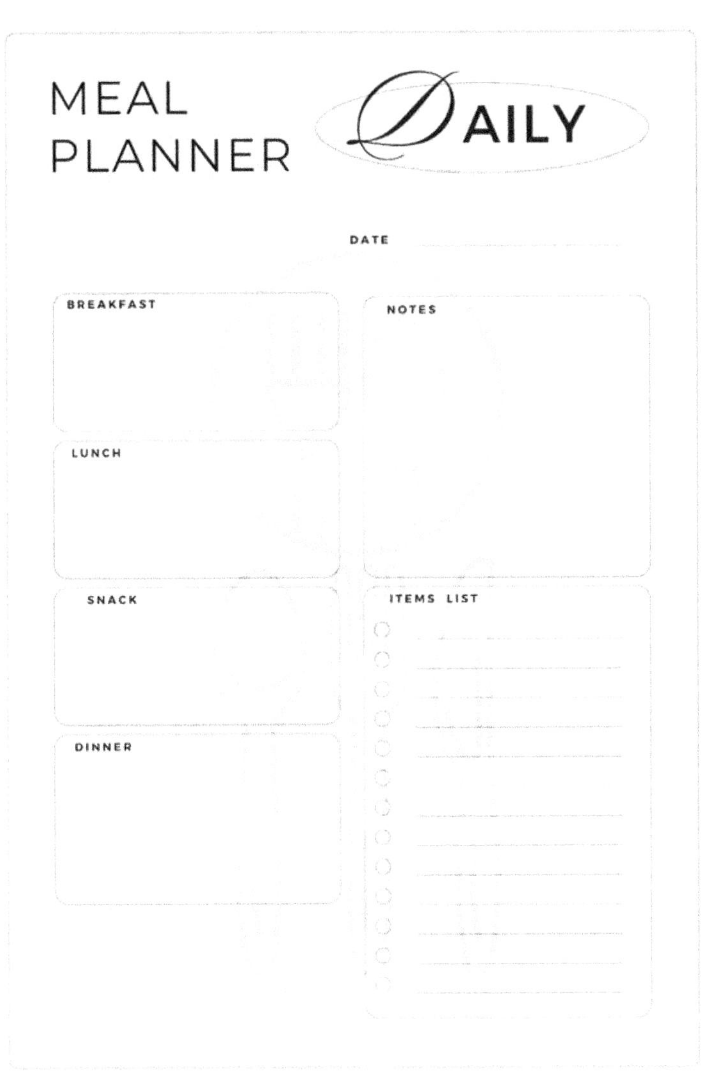

MEAL PLANNER

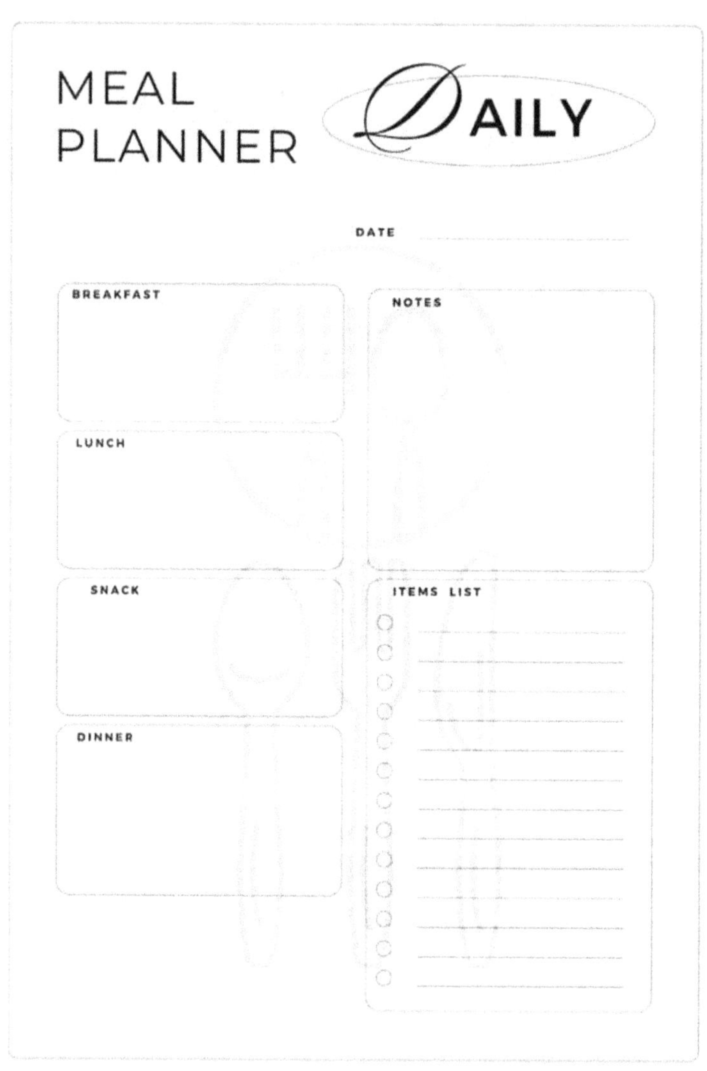

DAILY

DATE

BREAKFAST

NOTES

LUNCH

SNACK

ITEMS LIST

DINNER

MEAL PLANNER

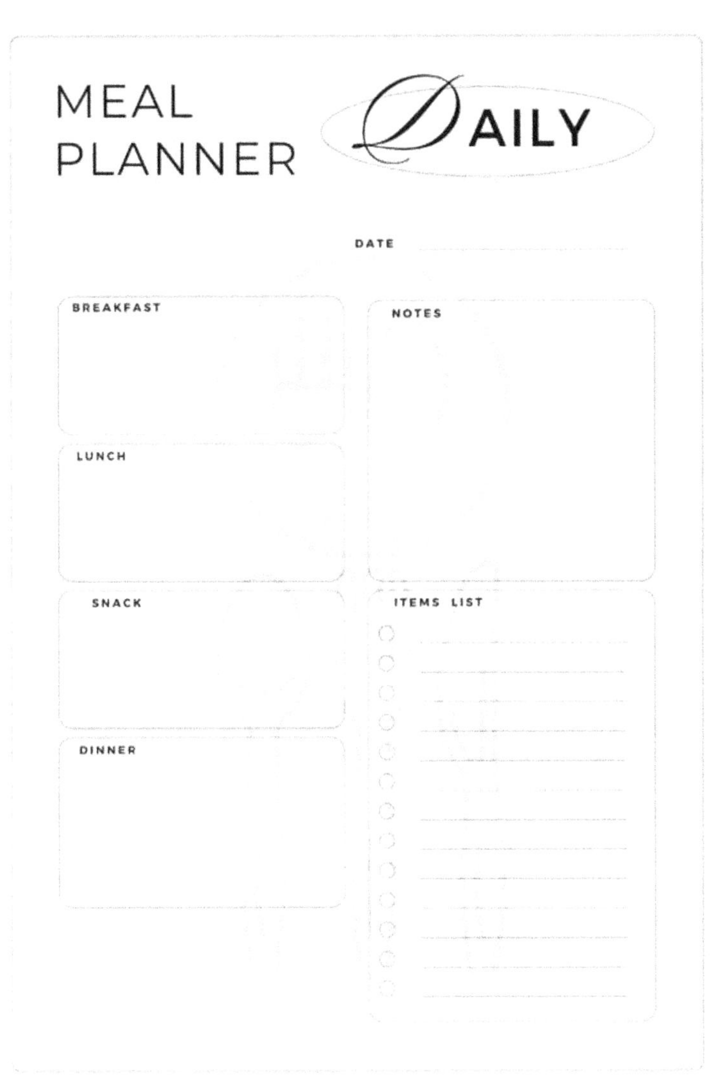

MEAL PLANNER

*D*AILY

DATE

BREAKFAST

NOTES

LUNCH

SNACK

ITEMS LIST

DINNER

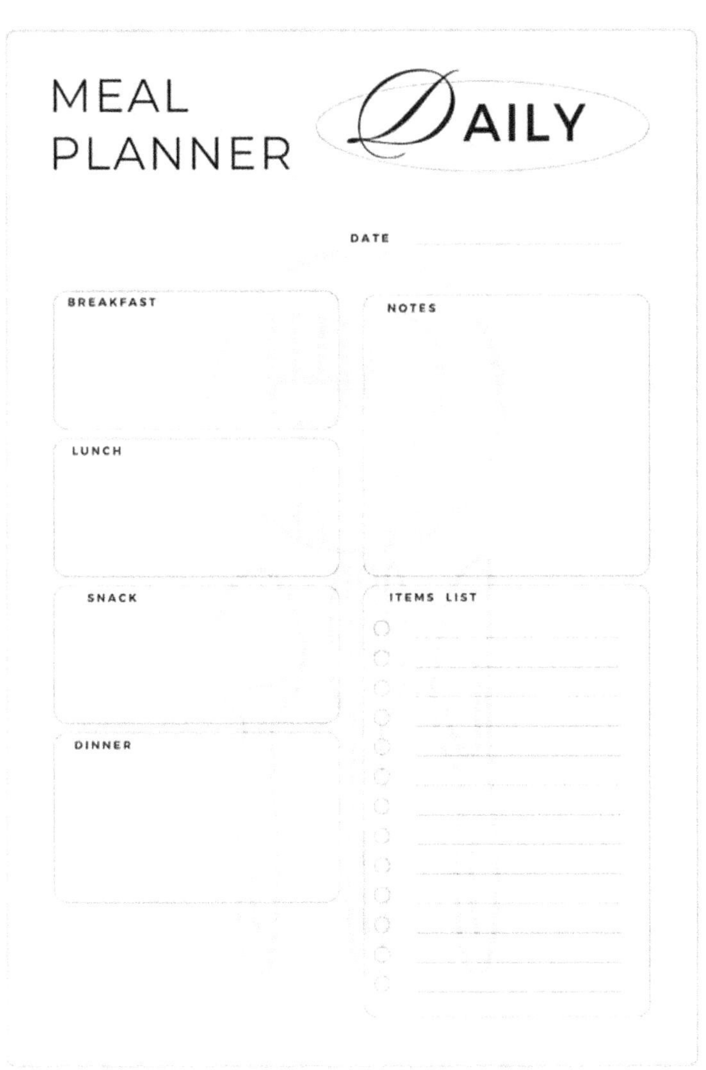

MEAL PLANNER
DAILY
DATE
BREAKFAST
NOTES
LUNCH
SNACK
ITEMS LIST
DINNER

MEAL PLANNER

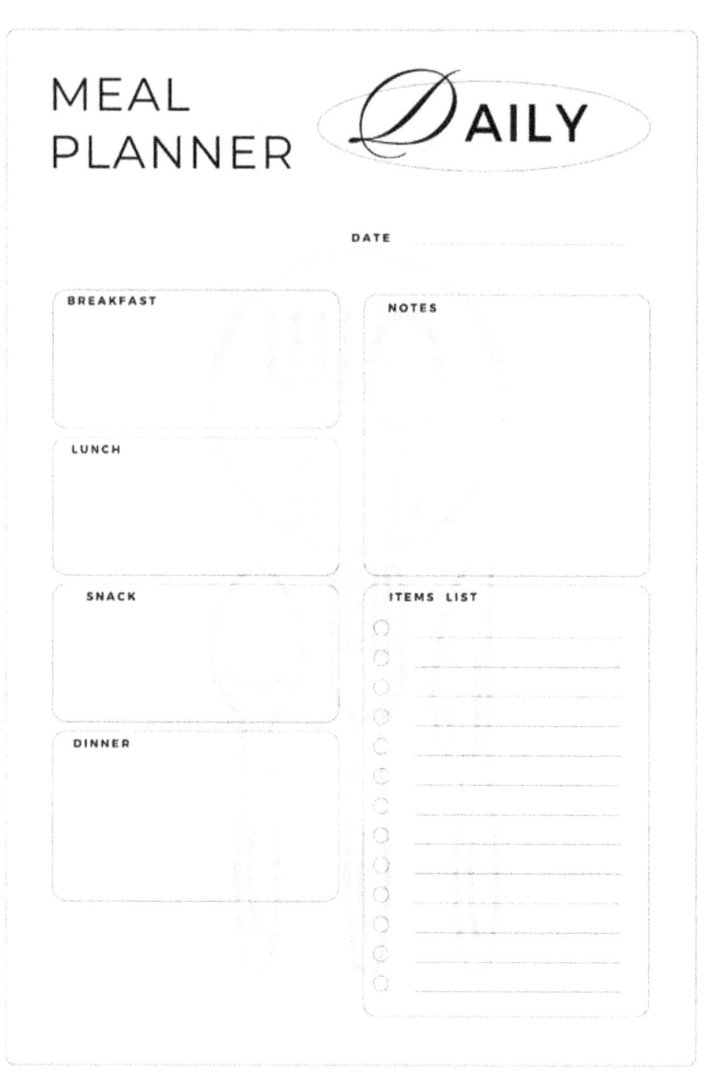

MEAL PLANNER

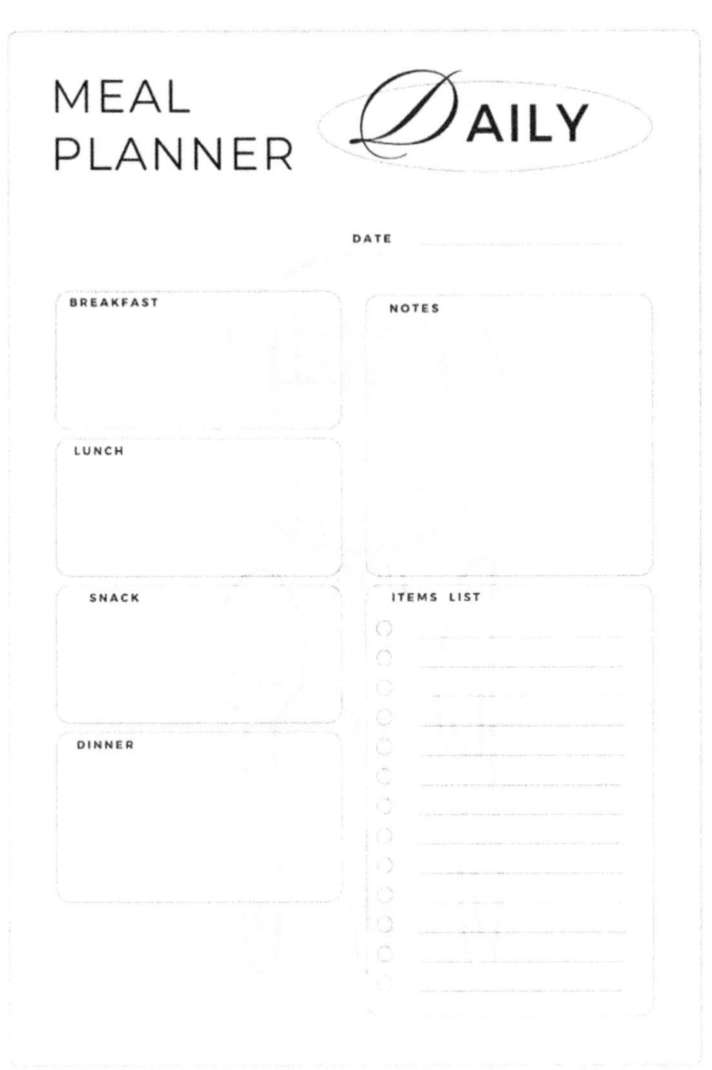

MEAL PLANNER $\mathcal{D}$AILY

DATE

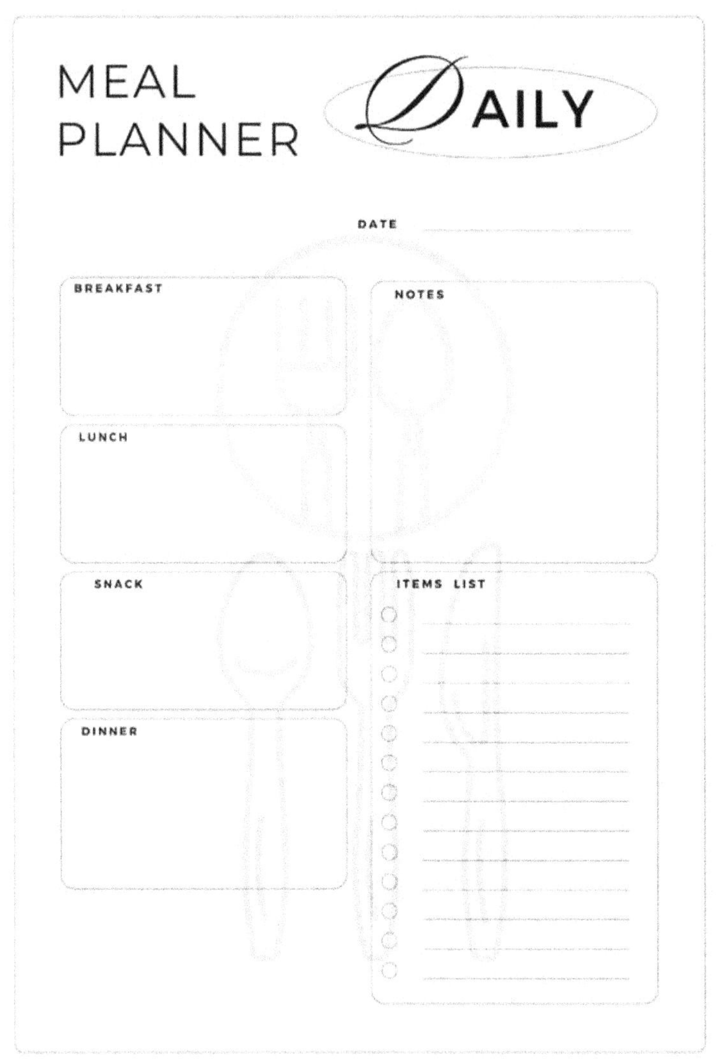

BREAKFAST

LUNCH

SNACK

DINNER

NOTES

ITEMS LIST